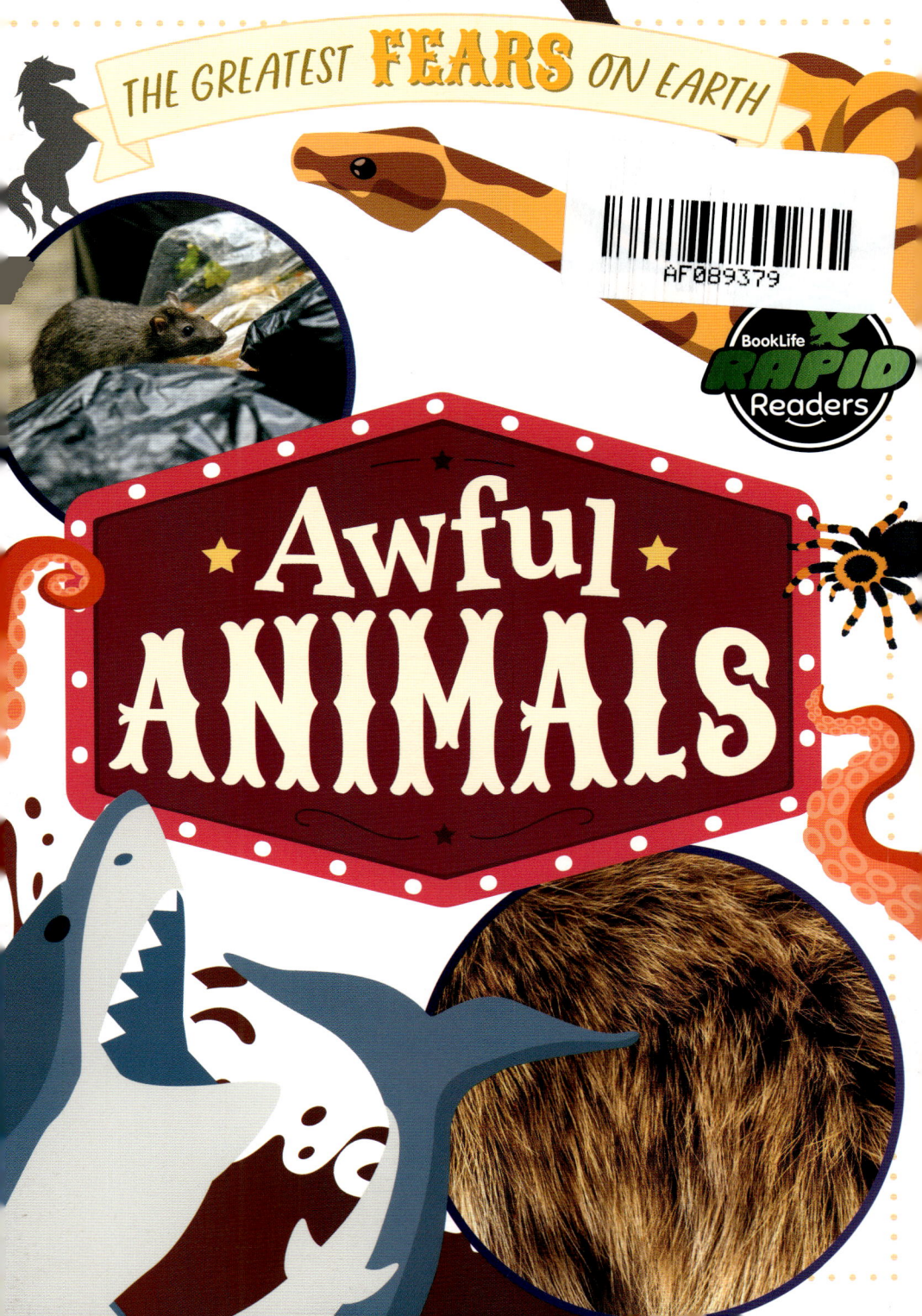

BookLife
PUBLISHING

©2023
BookLife Publishing Ltd.
King's Lynn, Norfolk
PE30 4LS, UK

All rights reserved.
Printed in China.

A catalogue record for this book is available from the British Library.

ISBN: 978-1-80505-027-8

Written by:
John Wood
Adapted by:
Noah Leatherland
Edited by:
Kirsty Holmes
Designed by:
Jasmine Pointer

All facts, statistics, web addresses and URLs in this book were verified as valid and accurate at time of writing. No responsibility for any changes to external websites or references can be accepted by either the author or publisher.

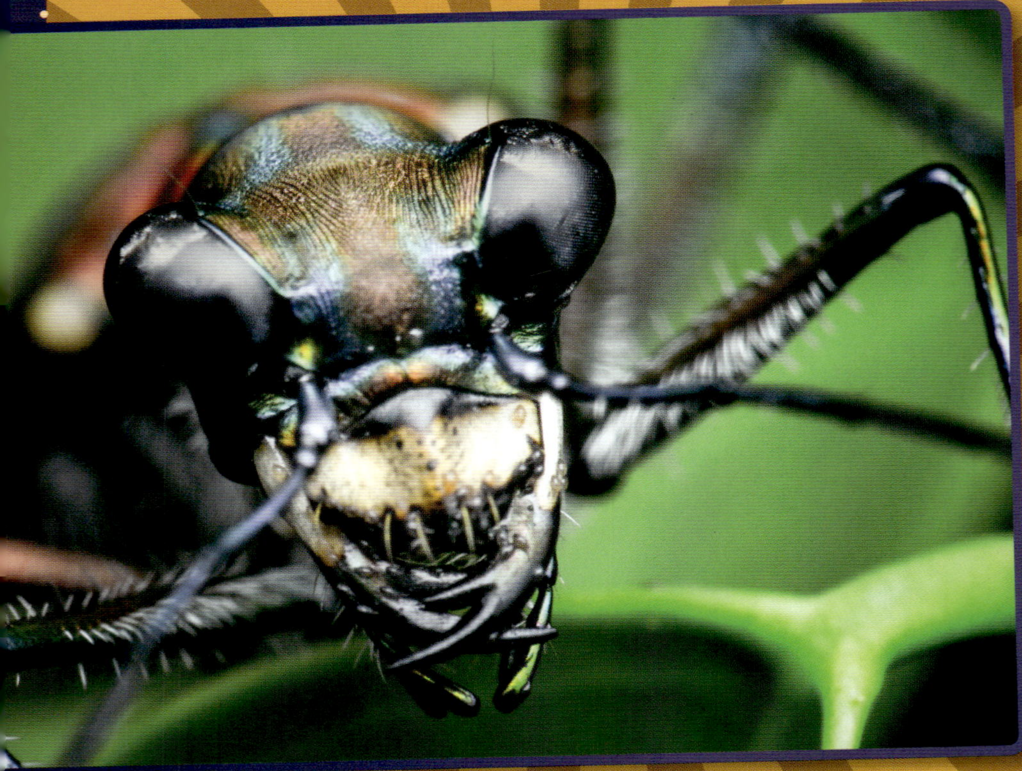

Photo Credits

Images are courtesy of Shutterstock.com. With thanks to Getty Images, Thinkstock Photo and iStockphoto.
RECURRING – pikepicture, kantimar kongjaidee, MagicMary. COVER – SpicyTruffel, Chanawat Jaiya, KittyVector, Svetsol, Vera Larina, Dalhazz, julio chaniago 76, Magicleaf, podtin. 4–5 – maxim ibragimov, sicegame. 6–7 – Kurit afshen, SpicyTruffel. 8–9 – Calvin Ang, Muangsatun, Kert, VectorShow. 10–11 – Studio 37, pirita, VectorPlotnikoff. 12–13 – Giovanni Cancemi, OlegRi. 14–15 – Sergey Uryadnikov, Willyam Bradberry, Gaslop. 16–17 – Scott E Read, oksana2010, Simply Amazing. 18–19 – Adwo, isarescheewin, Edge Creative. 20–21 – M Rose, Nadya_Art, Unknown Author, Public domain, via Wikimedia Commons. 22–23 – GOLFWORA, jekjob, LinaOro. 24–25 – Fehmiu Roffytavare, Fehmiu Roffytavare, Svetsol. 26–27 – Eric Isselee, Contes de fee, TigerStocks. 28–29 – clickit, Rudmer Zwerver, Photoongraphy.

CONTENTS

Words that look like this are explained in the glossary on page 31.

Page 4 Welcome to the Show!
Page 6 Scary Snakes
Page 8 Creepy Crawlies
Page 10 Horrid Horses
Page 12 The Science of Fear
Page 14 Shark Attack!
Page 16 Frightful Fur
Page 18 Our Guest Star
Page 20 Rotten Rats
Page 22 Shocking Shells
Page 24 Farm Fear
Page 26 Tarantula Terror
Page 28 Afraid of Animals
Page 30 Curtain Close
Page 31 Glossary
Page 32 Index

WELCOME TO THE SHOW!

"COME ONE, COME ALL! COME AND SEE SOME OF THE GREATEST FEARS KNOWN TO HUMANITY!"

We have all felt fear in our lives. But do you have a phobia? A phobia is a strong fear of something, such as spiders or flying.

People have phobias of all sorts of things. Some people have phobias of things where there is no real danger.

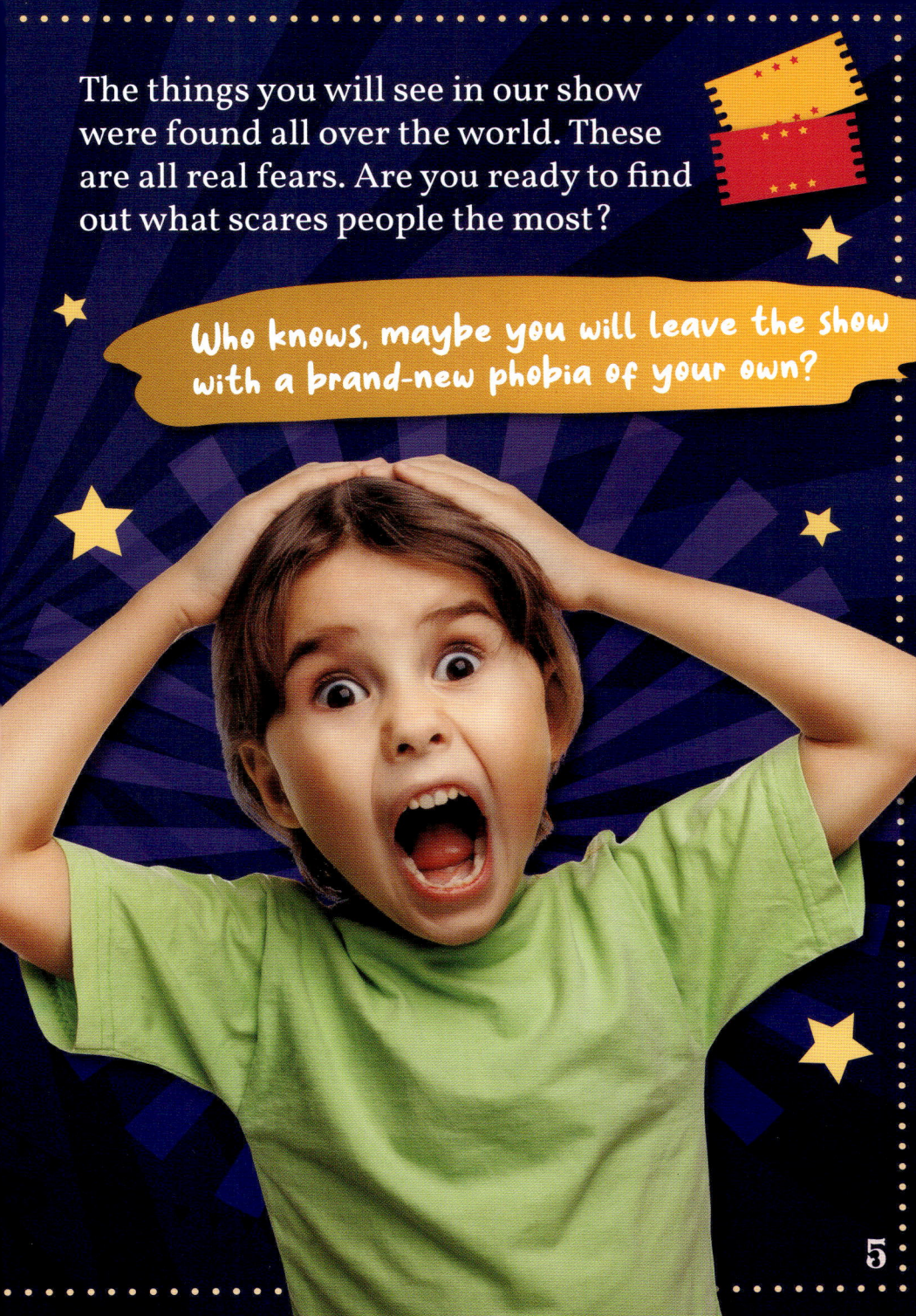

The things you will see in our show were found all over the world. These are all real fears. Are you ready to find out what scares people the most?

Who knows, maybe you will leave the show with a brand-new phobia of your own?

SCARY SNAKES

What is it about snakes that people find so scary? Is it the way they move? Maybe it is their speed? Sometimes they slowly <u>slither</u> across the ground. Sometimes they quickly <u>dart</u> at their prey.

Some people are afraid of how a snake looks. Snakes are covered in scales, and have sharp fangs, a pointy tongue and dark black eyes.

Some snakes are scary because they are dangerous. Some of them can **inject** an animal (or a person) with a deadly **venom**.

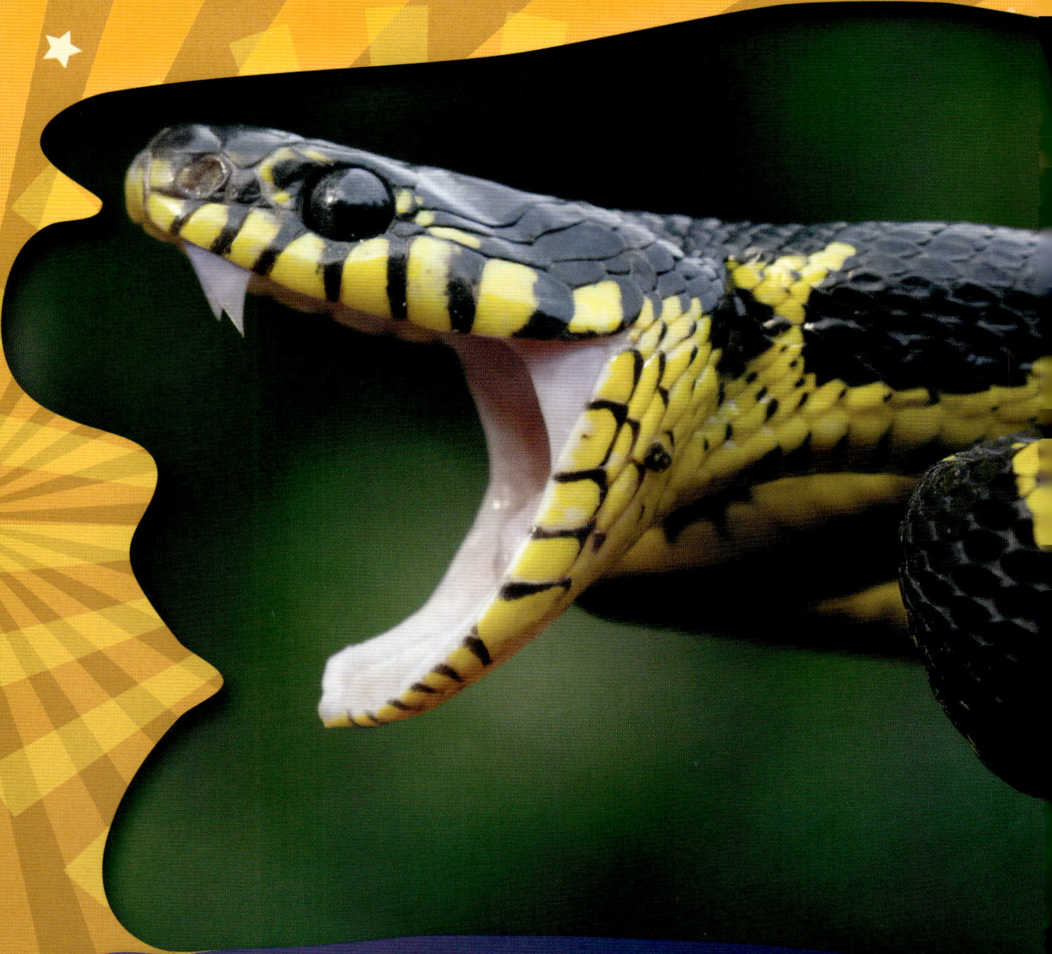

A lot of snakes are not dangerous, but that does not stop people being afraid of them. Are you afraid of snakes? What if one was slithering up your arm now?

CREEPY CRAWLIES

Even small things can be scary. How do you feel about bugs?

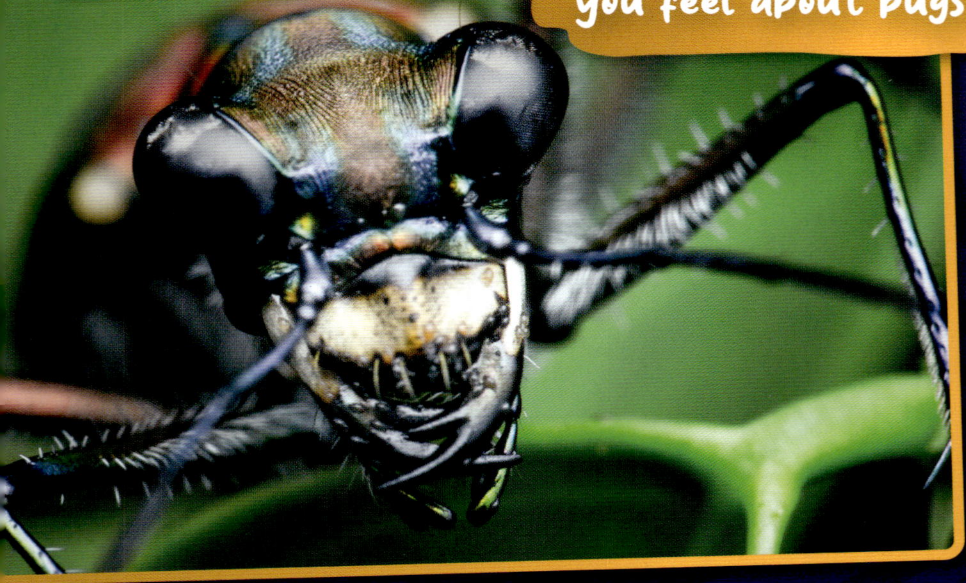

There are so many types of insects, and lots of things make them scary. Some of them buzz, some click and some we cannot hear at all. They might fly above our heads or crawl beside our feet.

You are never very far from a creepy crawly.

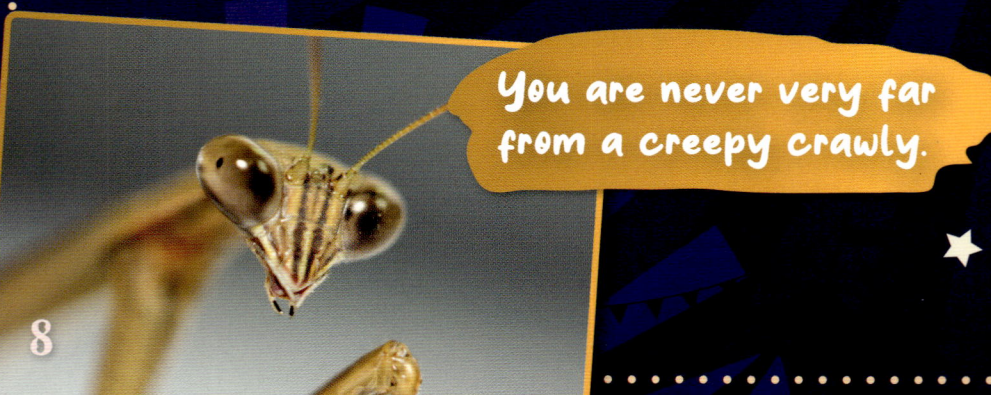

People do not like the way they look, the way they move or the tingly feeling of a bug crawling on them. Some people even think they feel insects on their skin even when there are none there.

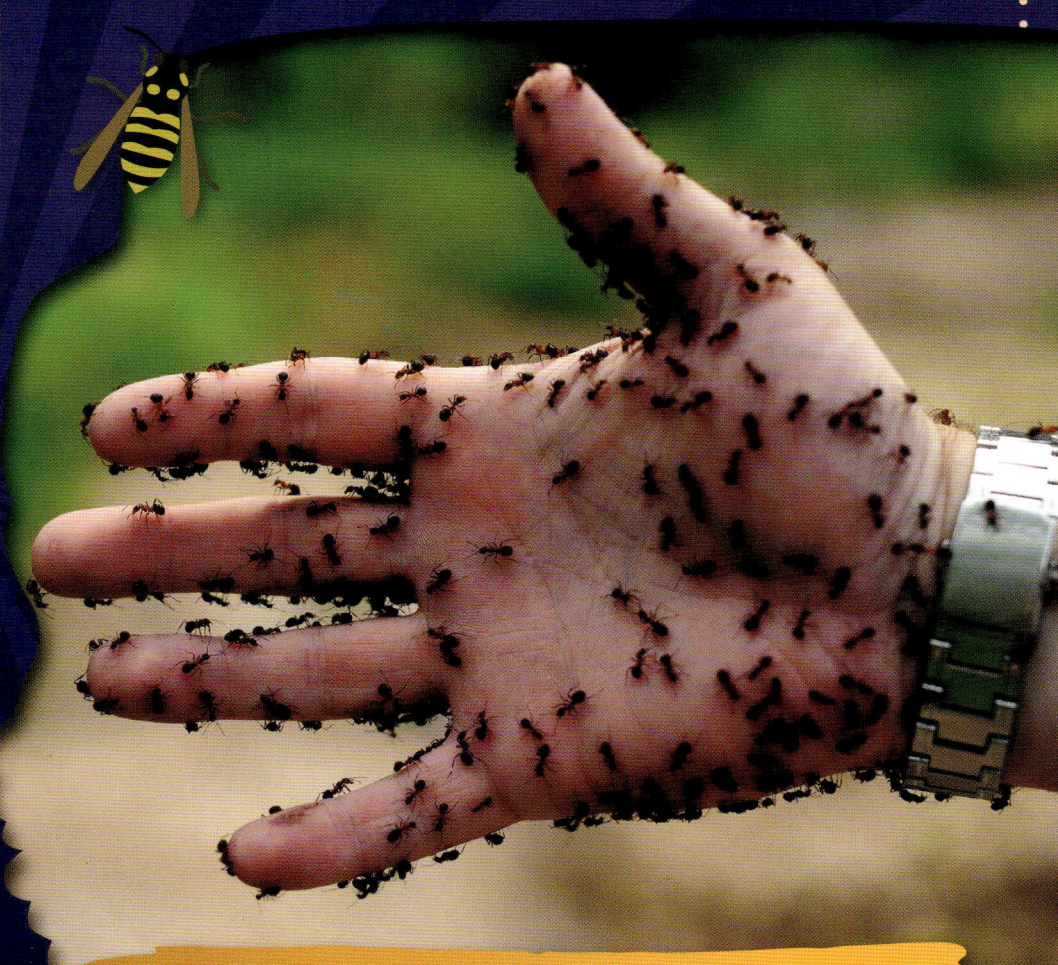

There are around 1.4 billion insects for every person on Earth. Who knows, perhaps there is a bug with its eyes on you right now...

HORRID HORSES

Some people love horses, but to others there is nothing scarier. Horses are big and strong. The biggest horse to ever live was 2.19 metres tall. That is taller than most adults!

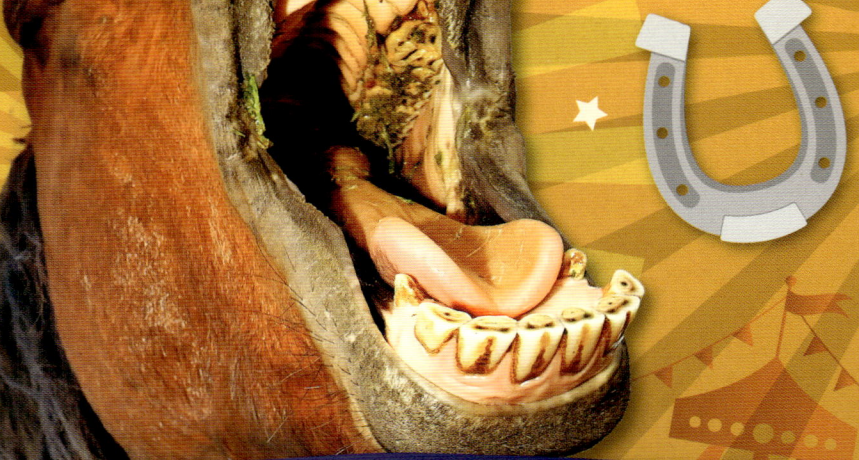

Horses are very powerful. You can see why some people are scared of them. Their massive yellow teeth are great for chewing their food. Imagine what they could do to a hand!

Not all horses are well behaved. Just because a horse has a saddle does not mean it is not wild at heart. Their strong hooves and muscles mean a horse's kick can be very dangerous.

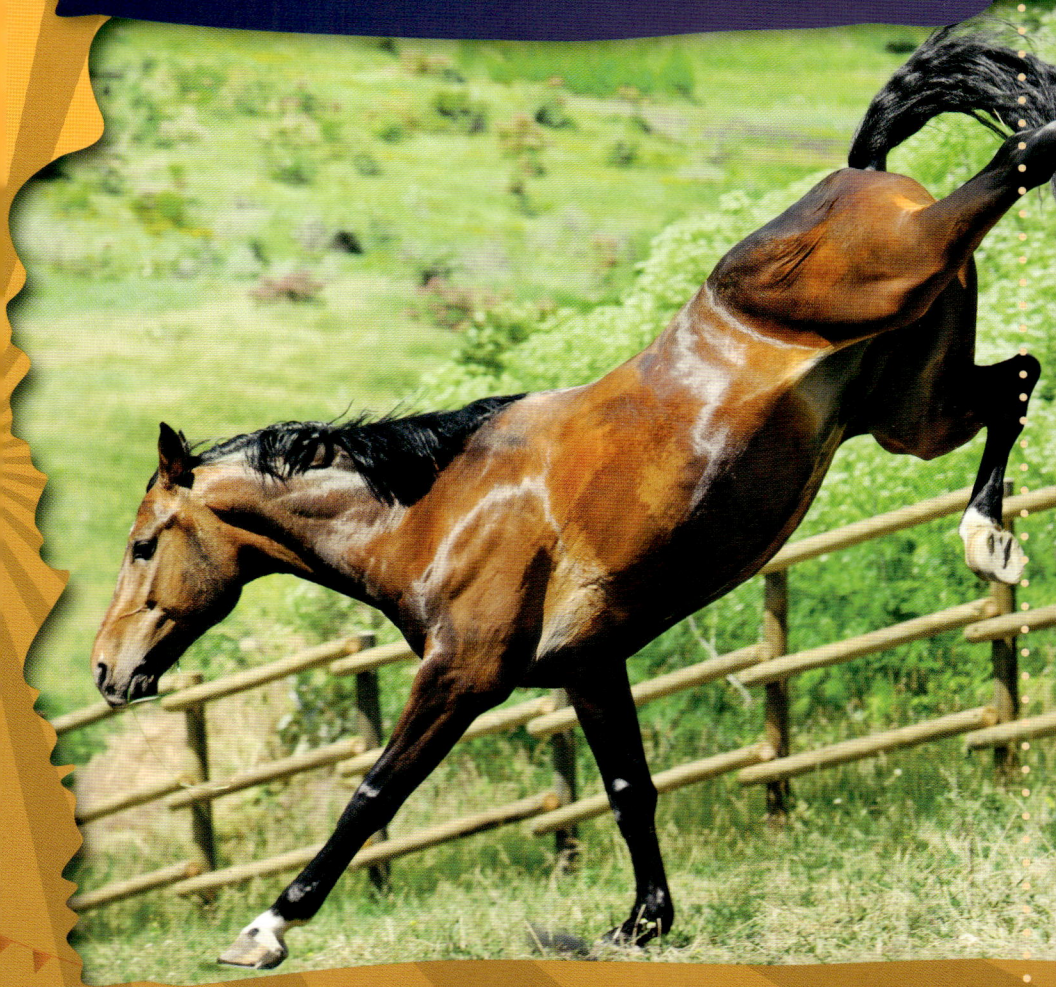

People with a phobia of horses might also be scared of other animals with hooves, such as ponies, donkeys and mules.

THE SCIENCE OF FEAR

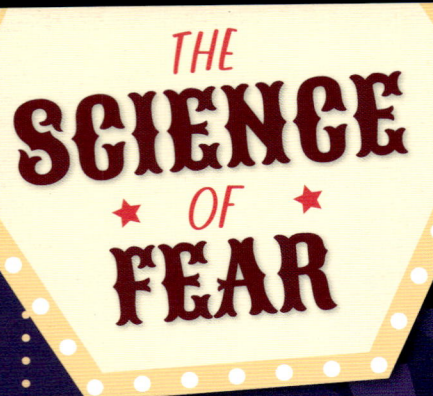

Your body has three <u>responses</u> when you are scared.

FIGHT
You might feel angry, and your muscles might tense up. You feel ready to lash out at anything dangerous.

FLIGHT
Your heart beats faster and your breathing speeds up. You are ready to run away and escape.

FREEZE
You feel like you cannot move or think. Scientists think this might be your body trying to play dead.

These <u>instincts</u> helped humans live in the wild thousands of years ago.

The fight, flight, freeze response is very important for humans. However, sometimes your body and brain get confused about what is dangerous. When you have a phobia, you get scared about something that might not be dangerous at all.

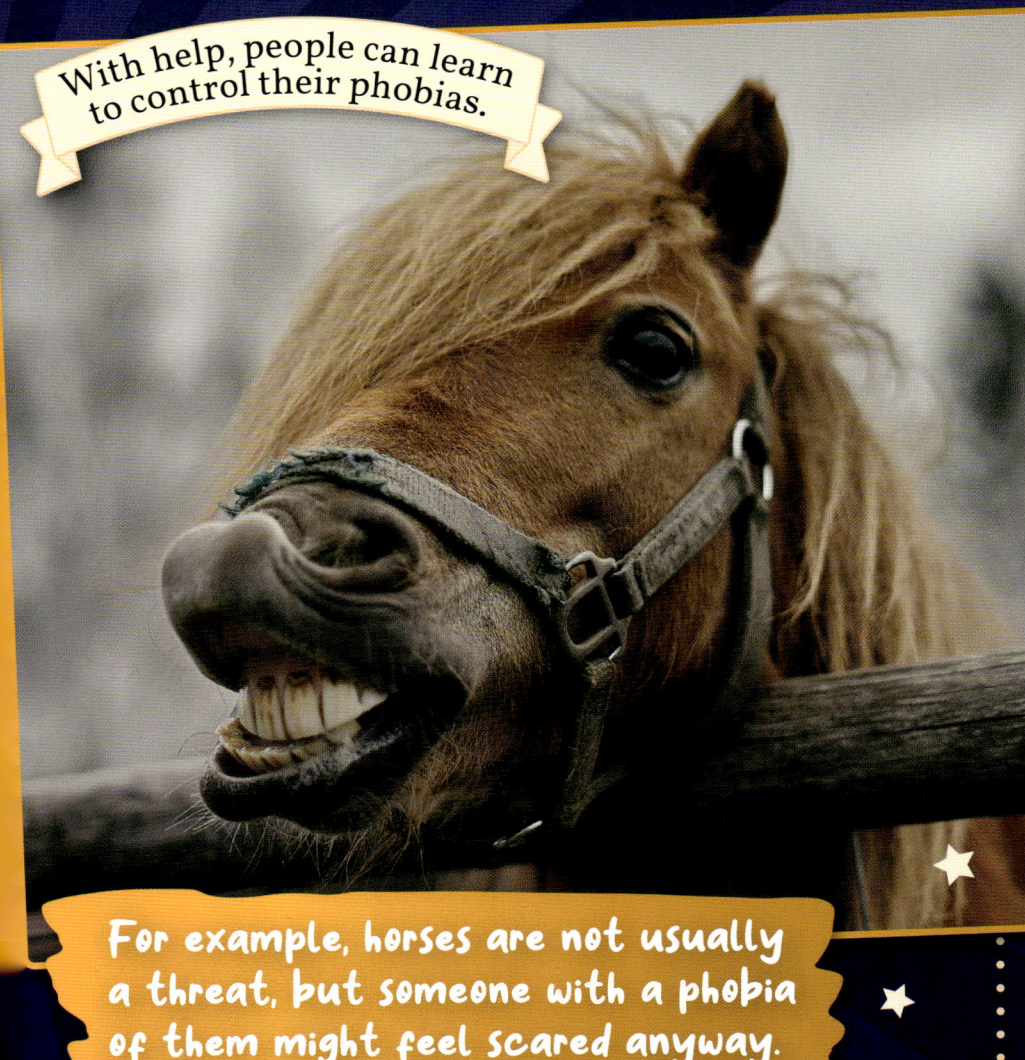

With help, people can learn to control their phobias.

For example, horses are not usually a threat, but someone with a phobia of them might feel scared anyway.

SHARK ATTACK!

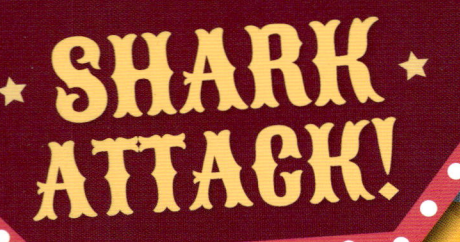

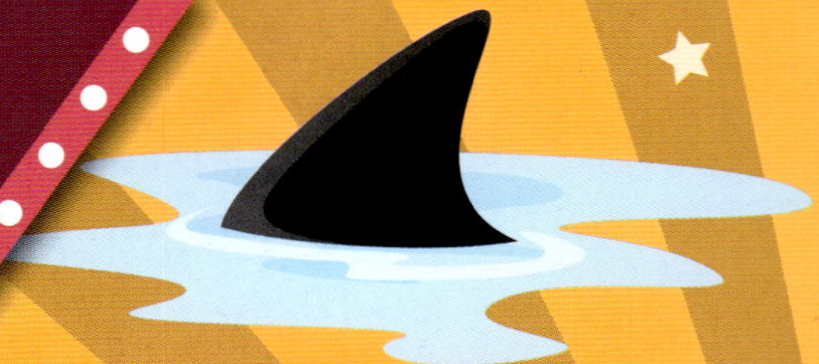

Deep underwater, giant sharks swim through the darkness. They are always looking for their next meal, following the smell of blood in the water.

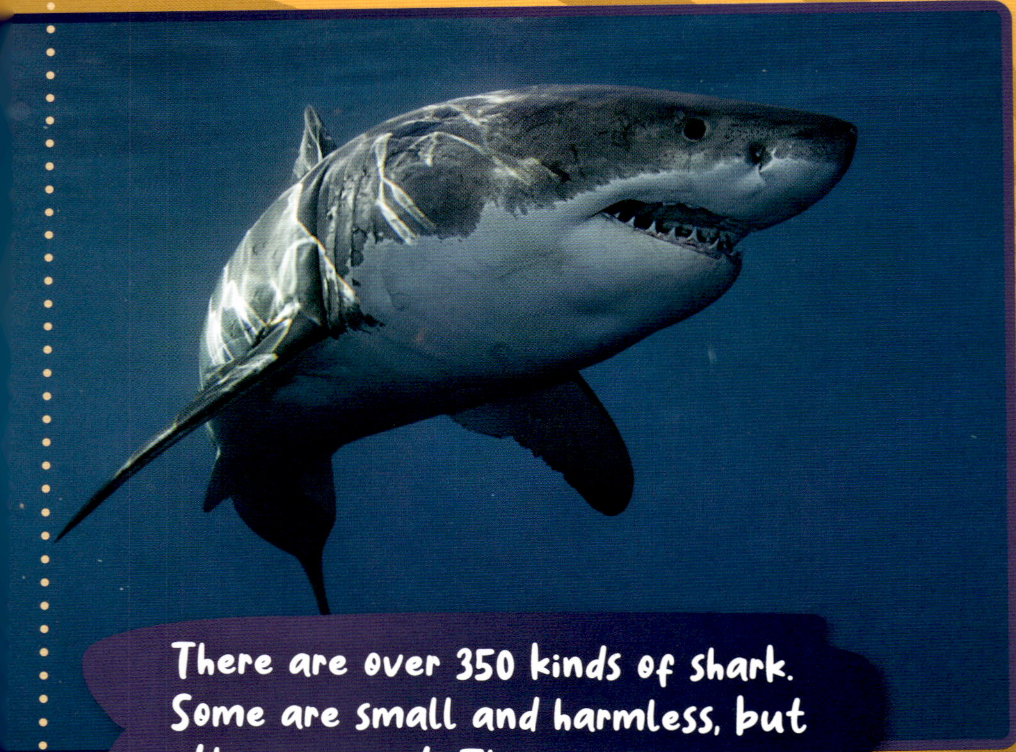

There are over 350 kinds of shark. Some are small and harmless, but others are not. They are some of the top predators in the oceans.

Now... Who is brave enough to jump into the shark tank?

Sharks have rows and rows of sharp, deadly teeth. When one falls out, another comes forward to take its place. All these teeth make sharks perfect hunters.

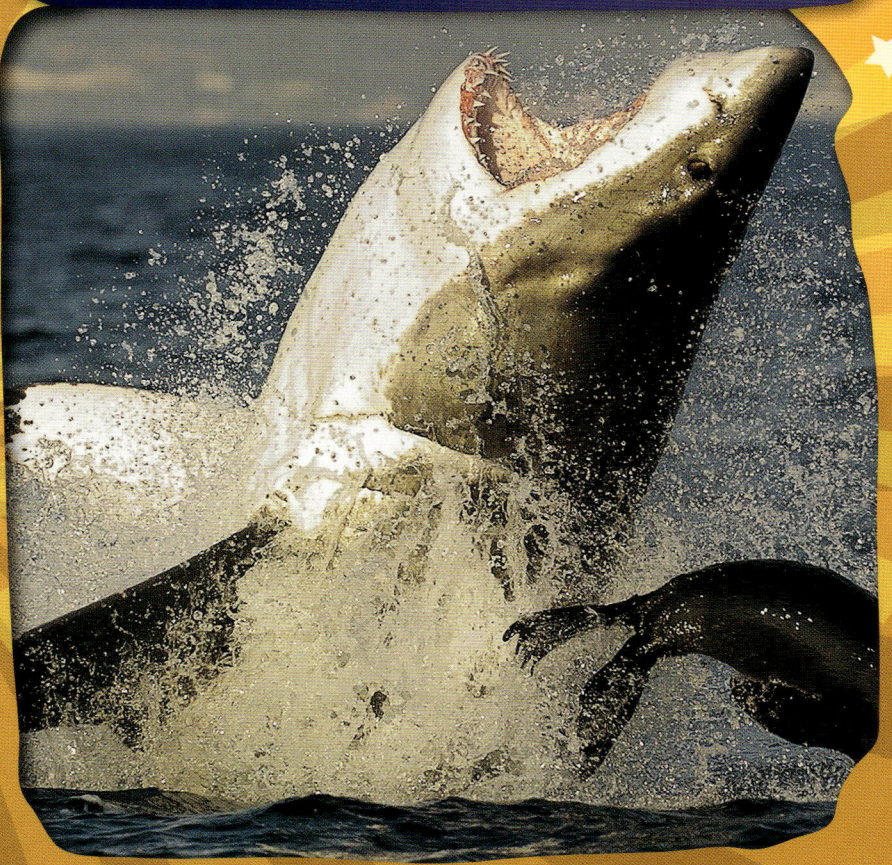

You are very unlikely to get bitten by a shark... but that should not stop you looking for shadows in the deep water. What would you do if you were swimming in the ocean and saw a shark? Would you be afraid?

FRIGHTFUL FUR

What will you see if you go into the woods? Maybe a bear? Or a pack of wolves? Those animals have lots of scary features, such as their sharp claws and teeth.

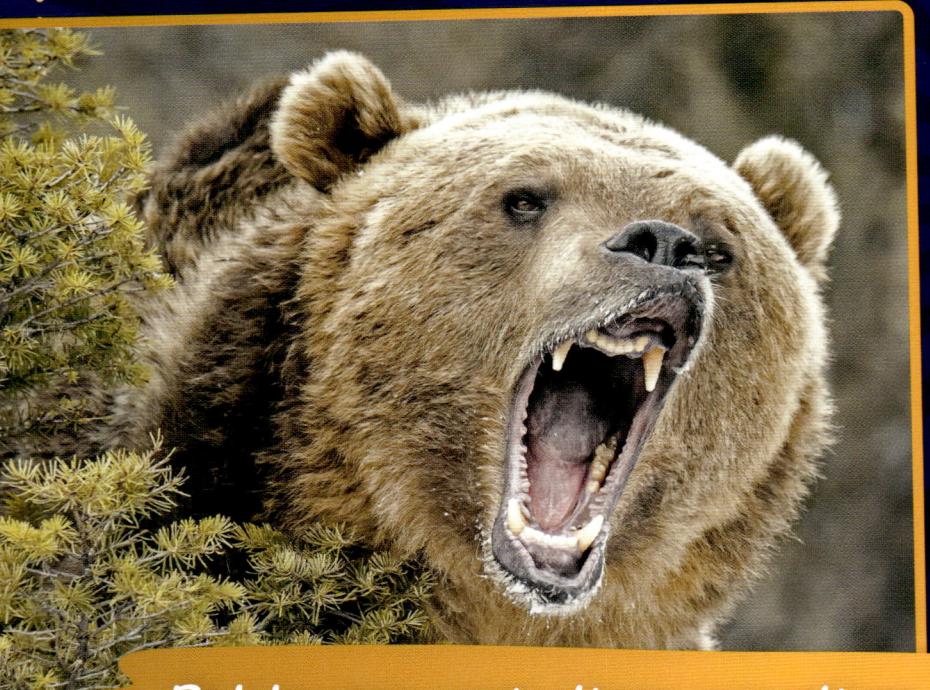

But to some people, there is something about them that is more frightening than that. For people with a fear of fur, there is nothing scarier than an animal's fur or skin.

The feel of fur is a big part of this phobia. How would an animal's fur feel? Soft or rough? Do your fingers get tangled in it? What about all the bugs and germs in their fur?

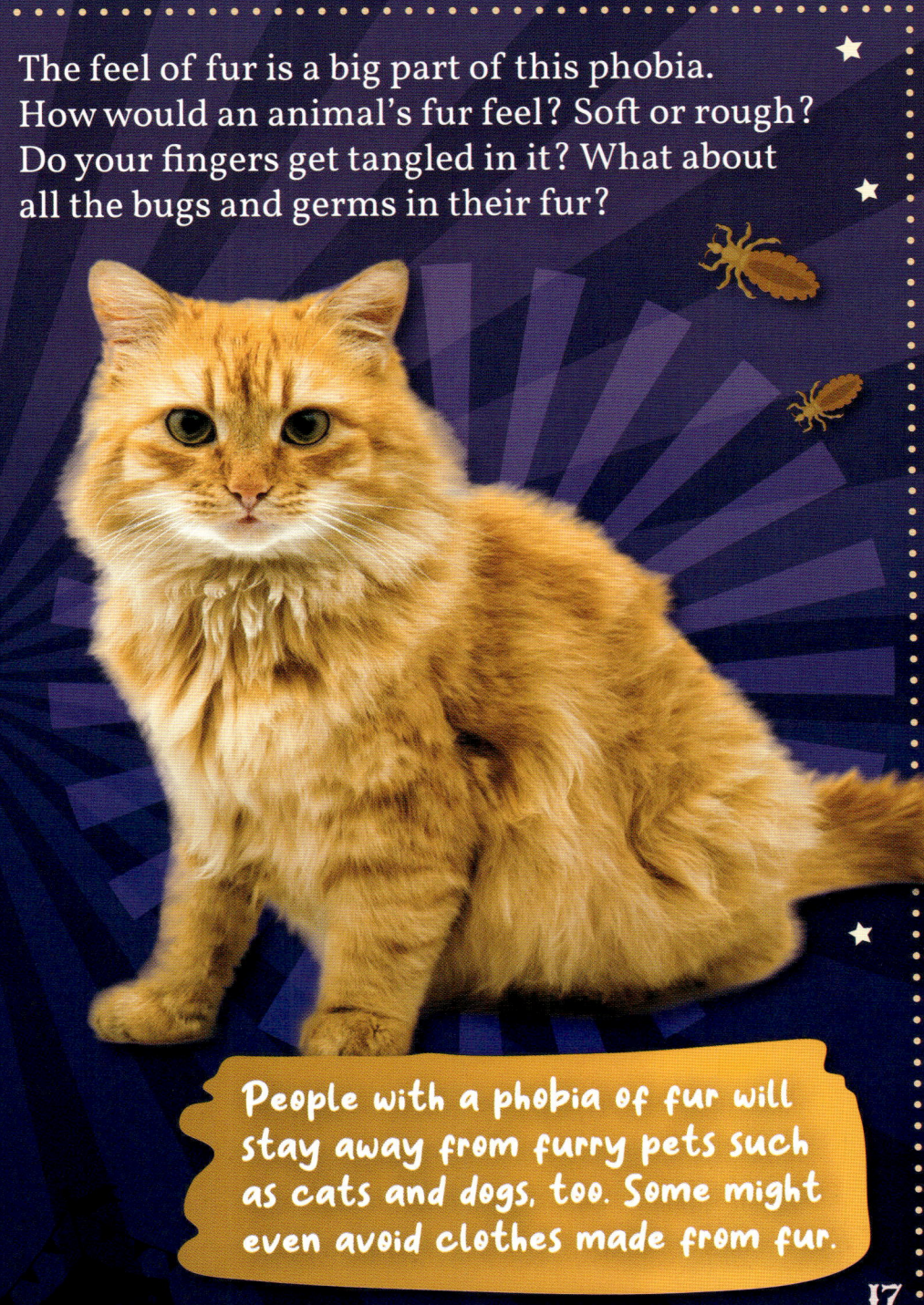

People with a phobia of fur will stay away from furry pets such as cats and dogs, too. Some might even avoid clothes made from fur.

OUR GUEST STAR

Genghis Khan was one of the most powerful warriors and leaders in history. He was born in Mongolia in 1162 and brought together all the tribes of the country.

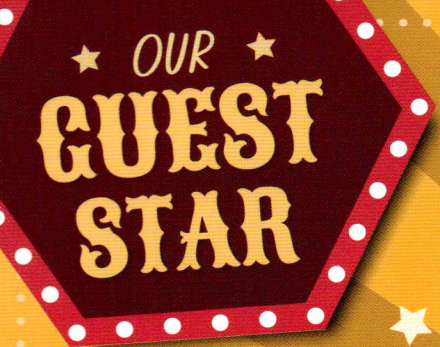

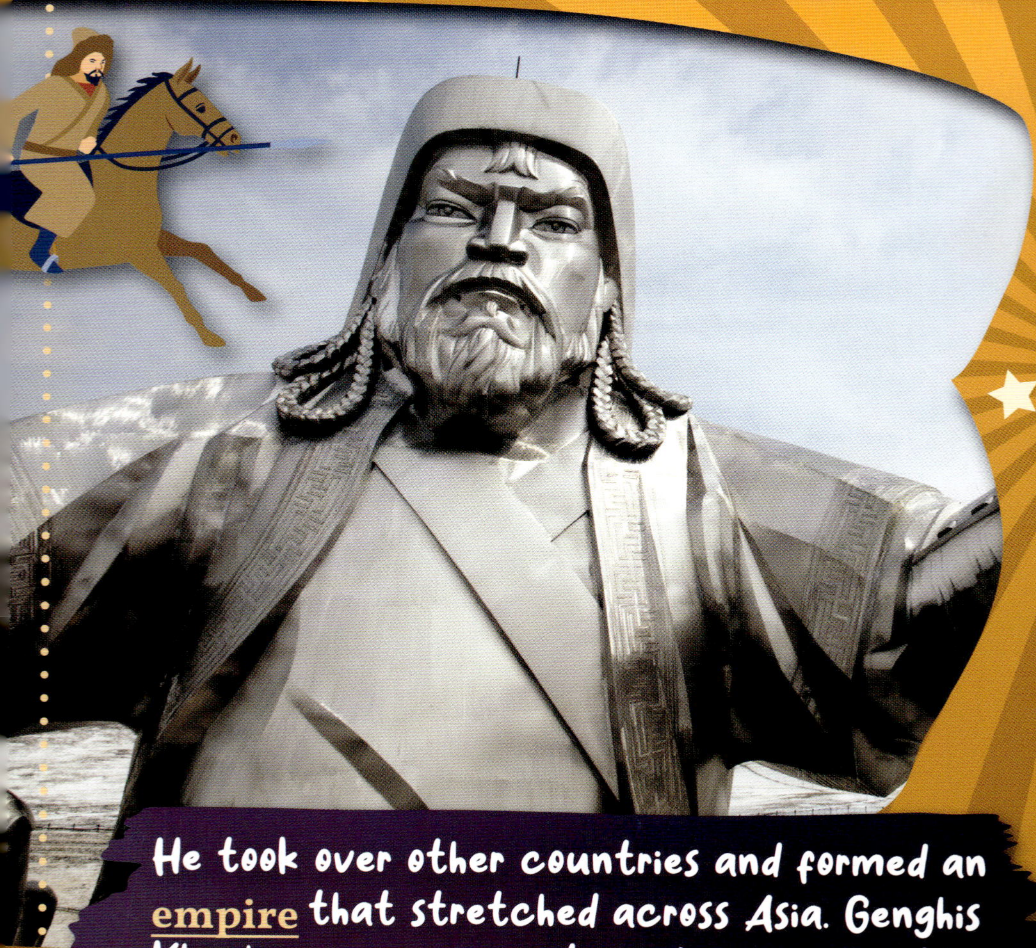

He took over other countries and formed an <u>empire</u> that stretched across Asia. Genghis Khan's armies were extremely scary, and his soldiers killed everyone they beat.

After taking control of so much land and winning so many battles, what could Genghis Khan have been afraid of?

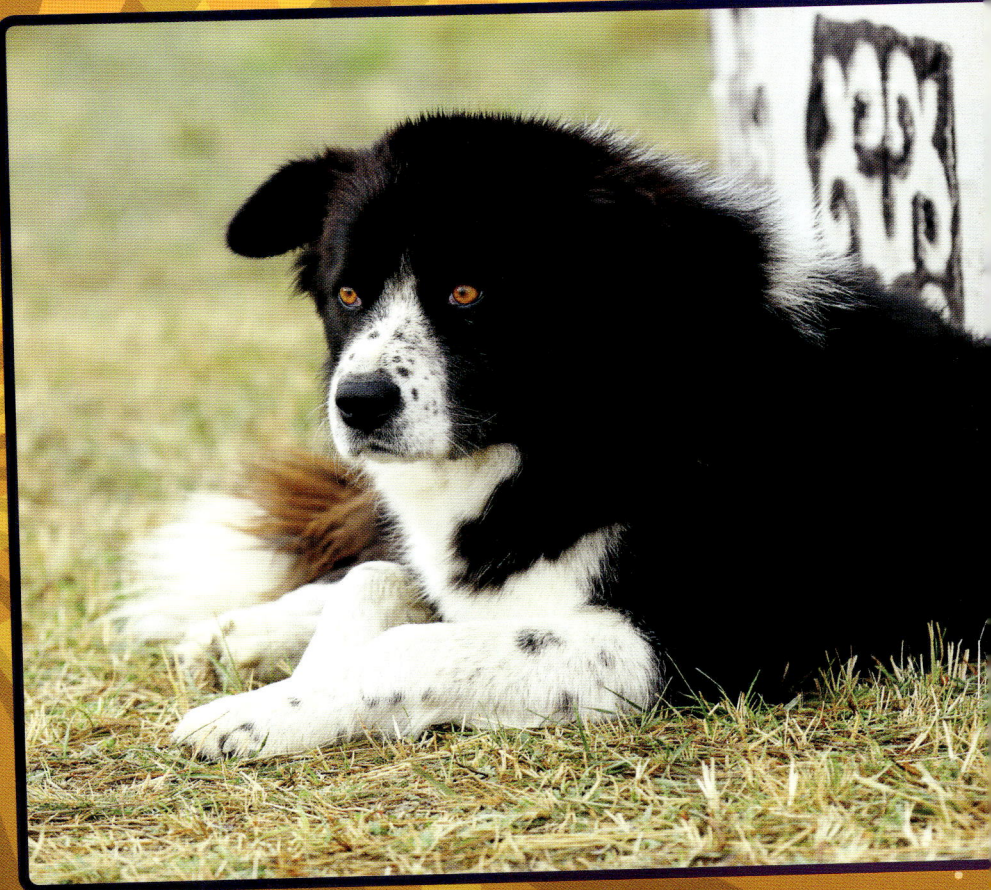

As it turns out, Genghis Khan had a phobia of dogs. To be fair to Genghis Khan, the dogs in Mongolia at this point in history were vicious and strong. That is why he called his **generals** his 'dogs of war'.

ROTTEN RATS

One species of animal has caused millions of deaths in history. They run through towns and cities, inside walls and into buildings. They can carry all sorts of diseases that can make people very sick.

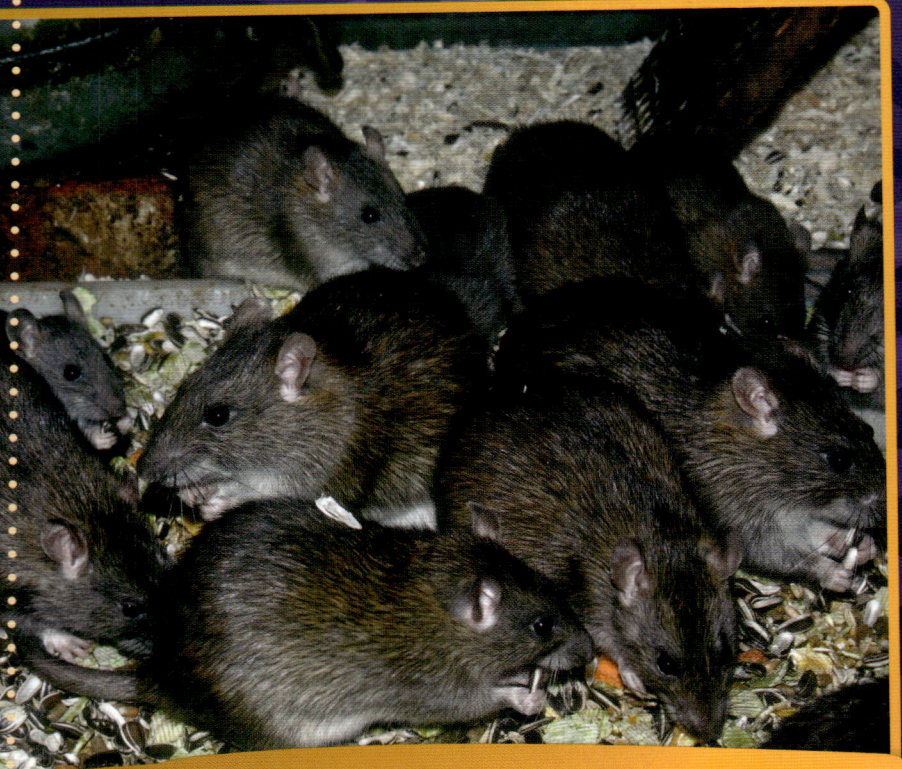

They are only small, but they terrify lots of people. They scurry and they squeak. They get everywhere. They are rats.

Although some people keep them as pets, rats can make some people's skin crawl. People with a phobia of rats might worry about what kind of nasty illness they might get from them.

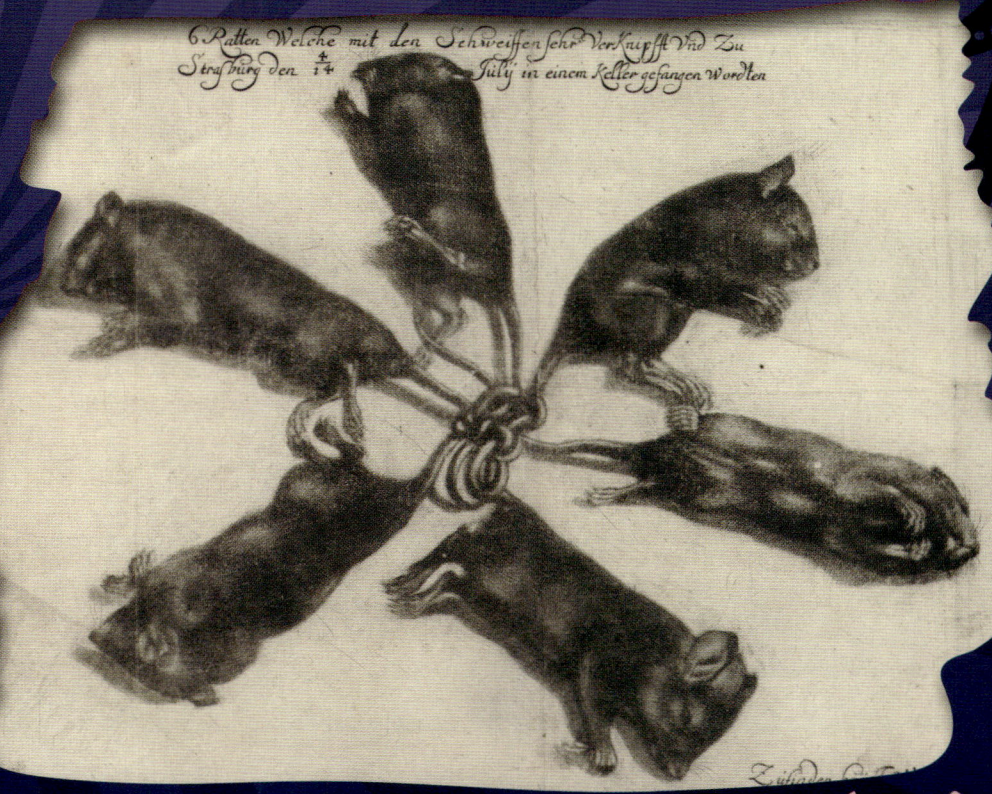

But the scariest of them all? The rat king. A rat king is when several rats get their tails tangled and become a savage ball of rats. Would you like to meet the rat king?

SHOCKING SHELLS

Shellfish are sea creatures with shells. Shrimp, crabs, lobsters and clams are all types of shellfish. They have some of the scariest body parts out of all the animals on the planet.

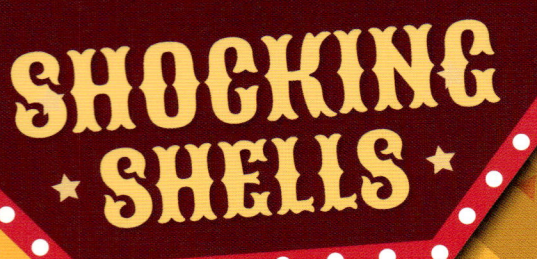

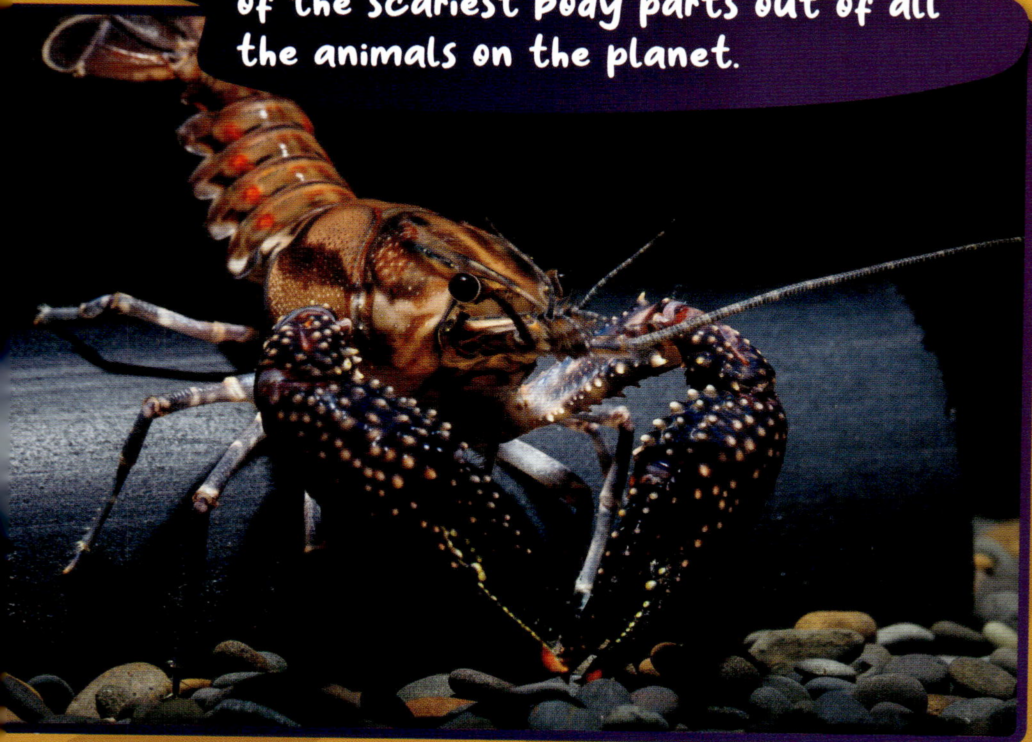

They live in deep parts of the sea, swimming and crawling along. They might have sharp <u>pincers</u>, spiky shells or long <u>antennae</u>.

Shellfish look strange – spiky, rough, slimy and gooey. They do not look too much different from aliens and sea monsters!

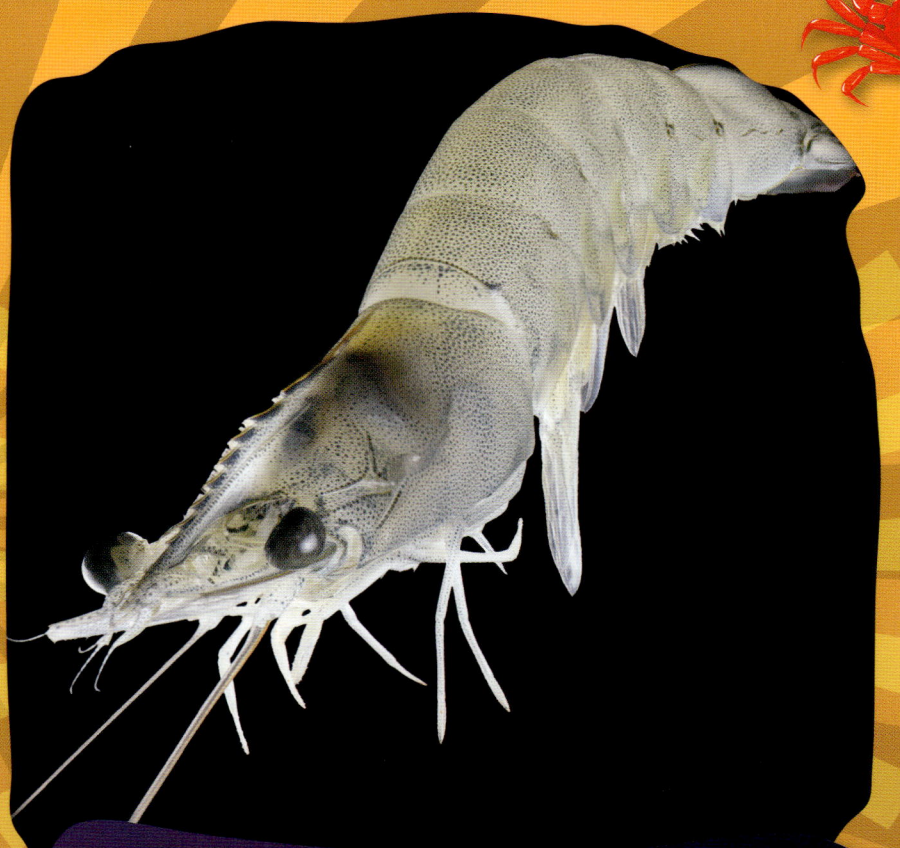

Many people like eating shellfish, but some are poisonous! For people with a phobia of shellfish, just the thought of eating one makes them panic. Shellfish are salty, slimy and slippery — would you eat one of these creepy sea beasts?

FARM FEAR

They are a small farm animal, but some people are really scared of them. Their heads bob and they make funny sounds.

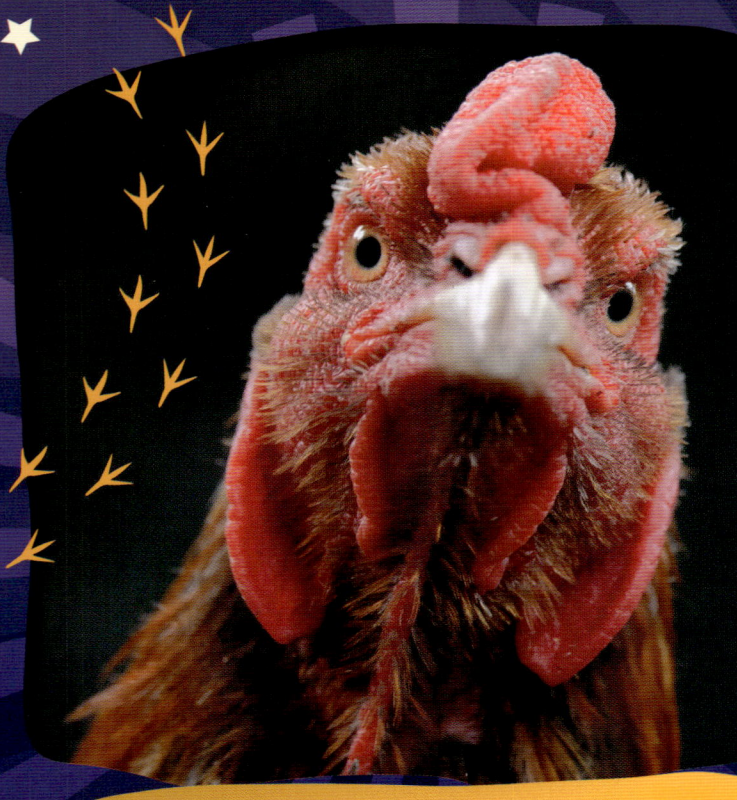

But they also have sharp beaks and claws. They have thin, scaly legs and little black eyes. If you are not careful they could come after you! They are the horrible, terrifying... chickens?

Do you ever look at a chicken and think they look familiar? Perhaps you think they look like a T. rex? You would be right – chickens actually **evolved** from dinosaurs! No wonder some people feel scared around them.

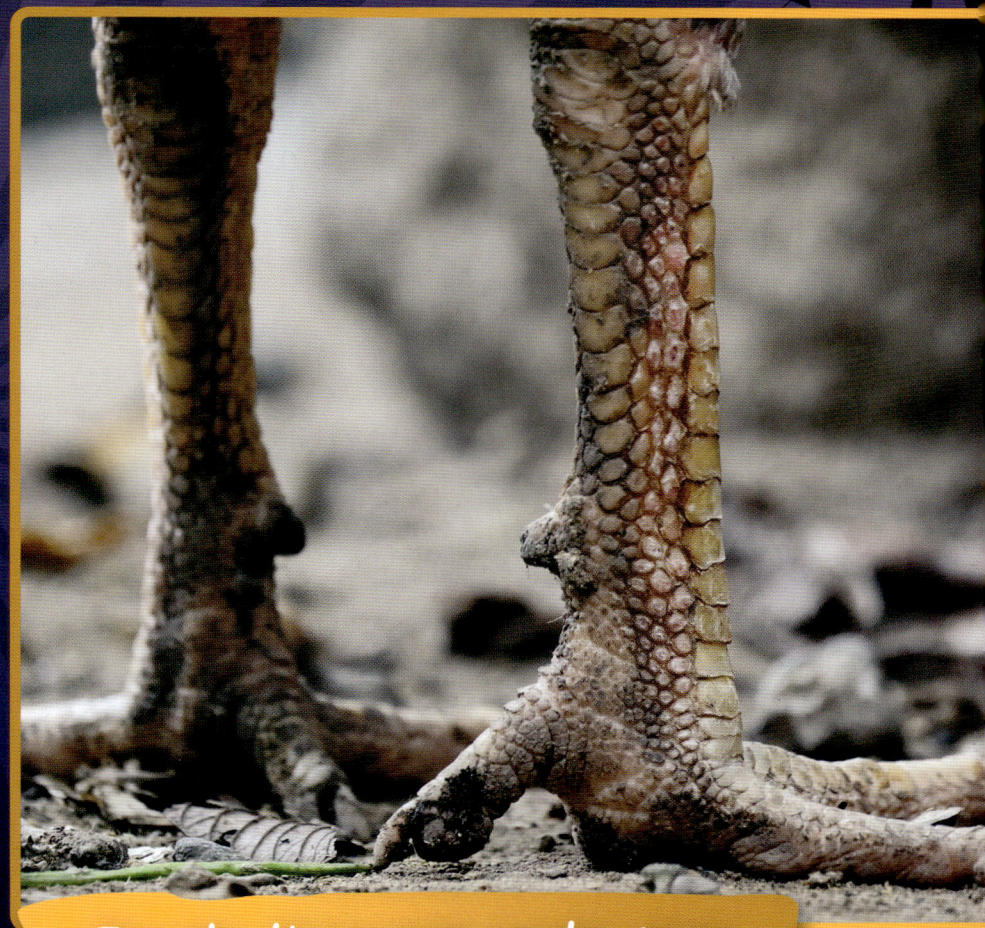

To make them even weirder, some chickens can survive a short time after having their heads cut off!

TARANTULA TERROR

And now, the most feared animal of all. They terrify children and adults all over the world — spiders! There are lots of things people do not like about spiders. Their bodies are covered in tiny hairs, all the way down their long legs.

They creep along walls and in dark corners. When you do spot one, they run away as fast as they can.

Just like snakes, some spiders can bite and inject other animals with venom. They do this with large, pointy fangs.

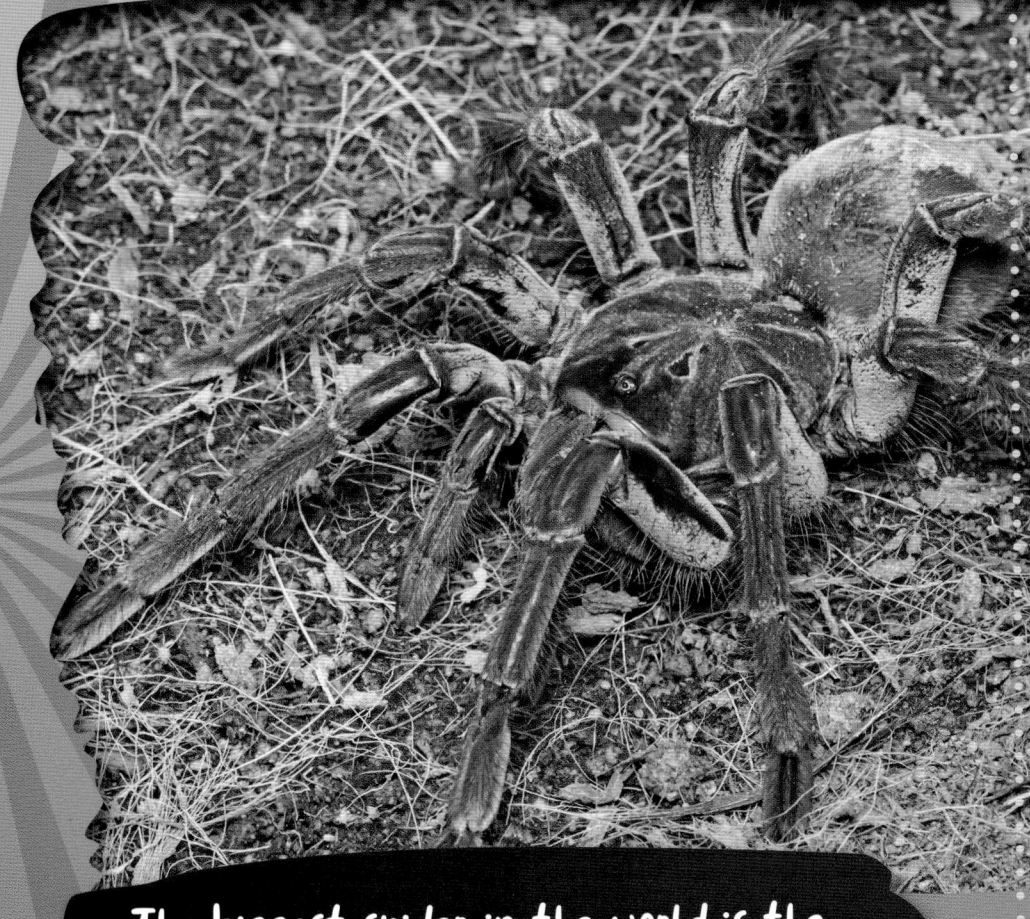

The biggest spider in the world is the Goliath Birdeater spider. Although some spiders have longer legs, the Goliath Birdeater has the biggest body, making it the heaviest spider in the world.

AFRAID OF ANIMALS

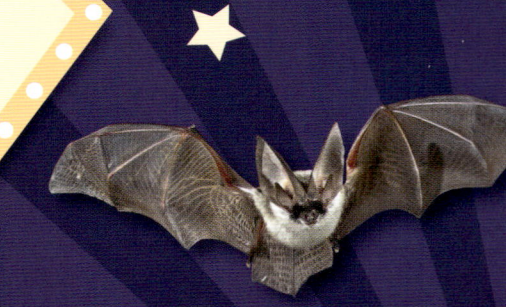

That is the end of our show! But do you have a phobia of one or more animals in the show? Is there a creature that makes you tremble all over?

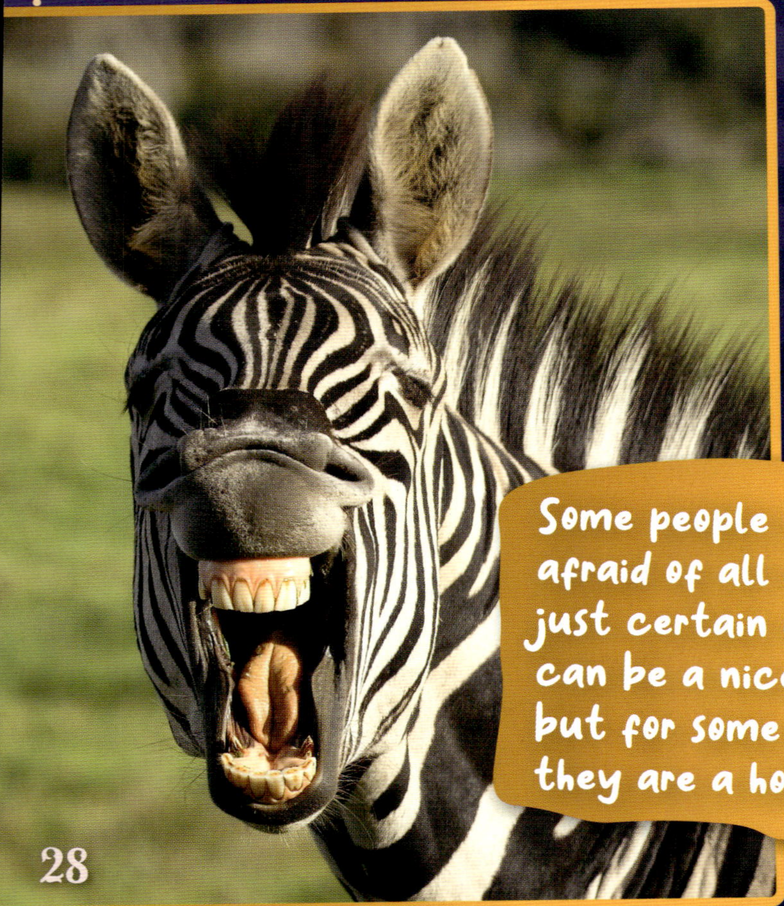

Some people might be afraid of all animals or just certain ones. Zoos can be a nice day out, but for some people they are a horror show!

Many animals have scary features, such as big teeth, sharp claws, horns, scales, speed, strength and more.

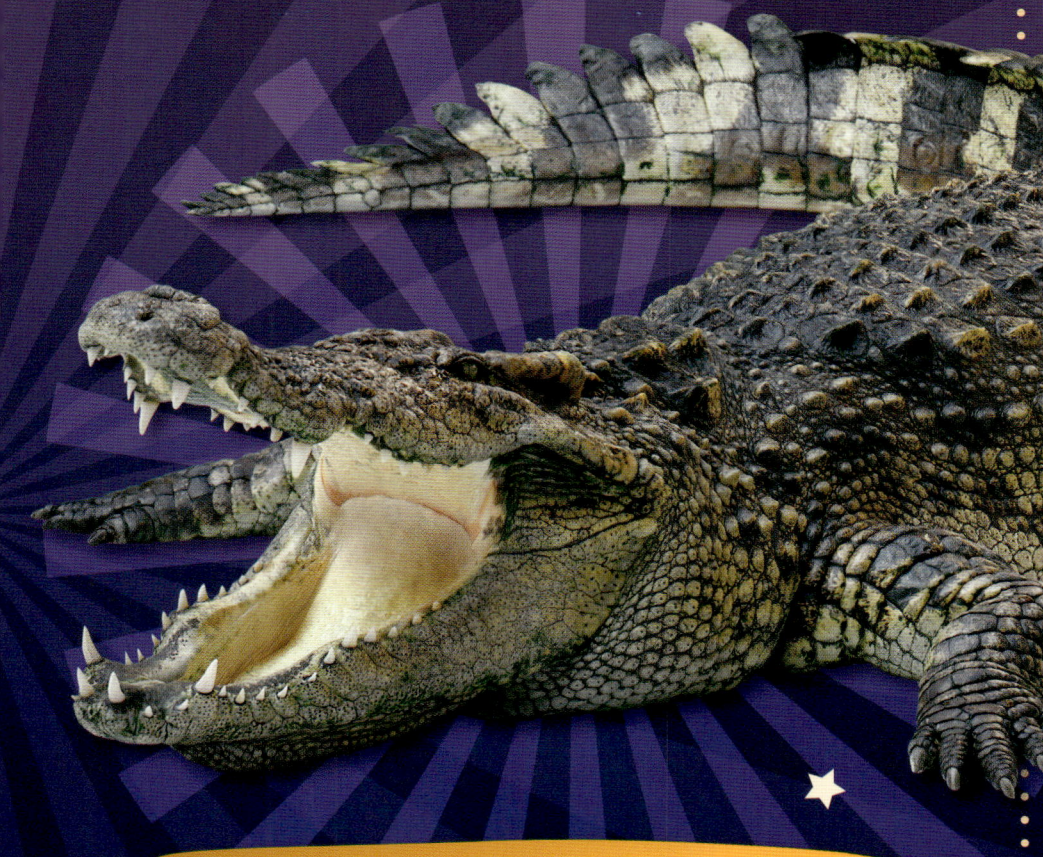

For some people, it is how different many animals are to us. We cannot talk to them. We cannot know what they are feeling or thinking. Who knows what is going on in an animal's head when it looks at you?

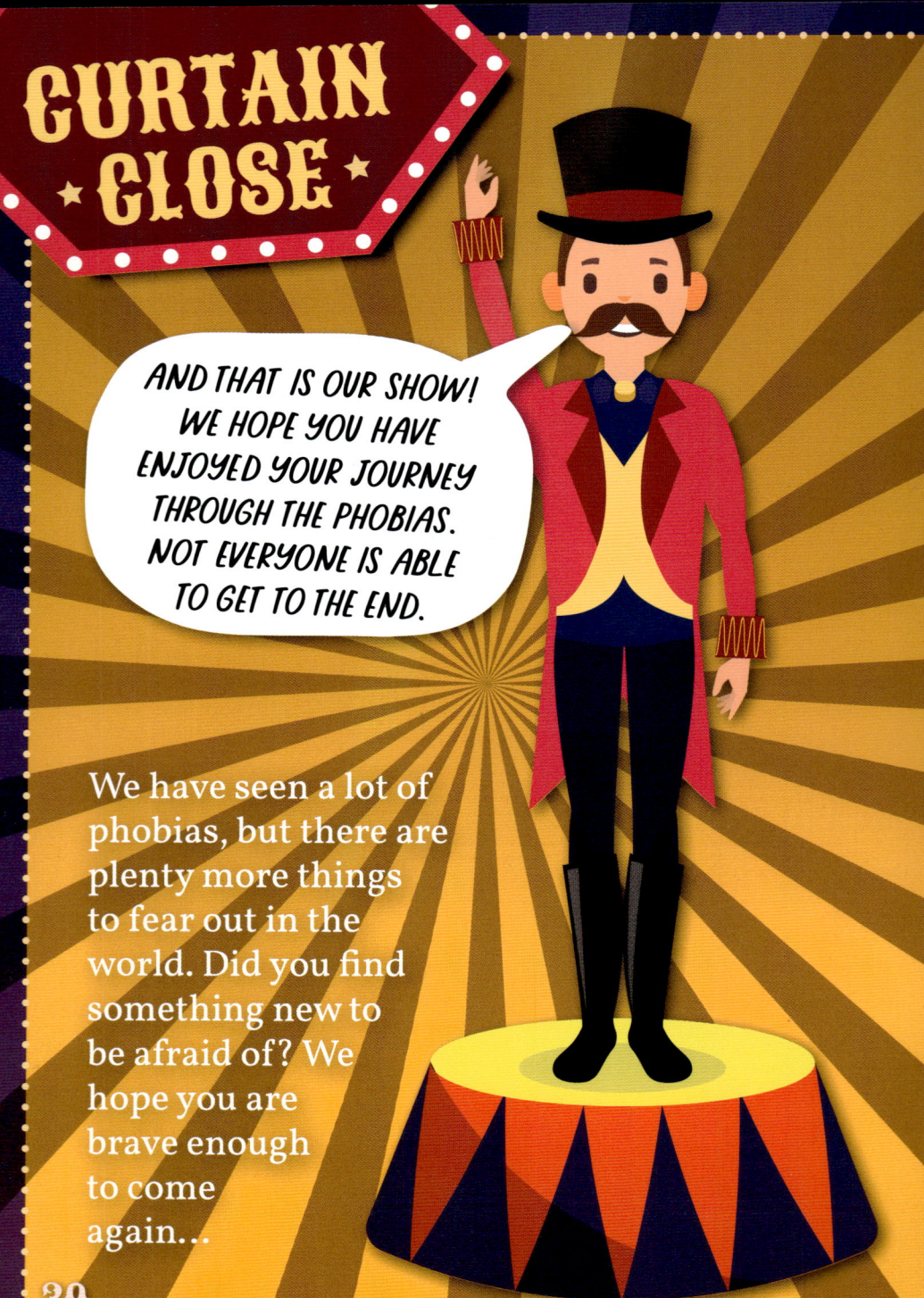

GLOSSARY

antennae — long, thin organs that come out of the head

dart — to move quickly

empire — a collection of countries with one ruler

evolved — changed over time

generals — people who lead armies

inject — to force a liquid into something

instincts — feelings of how to act

pincers — pairs of claws that grip things

responses — reactions

slither — to slide

venom — a harmful poison that enters the body through a bite or sting

INDEX

chickens	24–25	rats	20–21
dogs	17, 19	sharks	14–15
Genghis Khan	18–19	shellfish	22–23
horses	10–11, 13	snakes	6–7, 27
insects	8–9	spiders	4, 26–27

AN INTRODUCTION TO BOOKLIFE RAPID READERS...

Packed full of gripping topics and twisted tales, BookLife Rapid Readers are perfect for older children looking to propel their reading up to top speed. With three levels based on our planet's fastest animals, children will be able to find the perfect point from which to accelerate their reading journey. From the spooky to the silly, these roaring reads will turn every child at every reading level into a prolific page-turner!

CHEETAH
The fastest animals on land, cheetahs will be taking their first strides as they race to top speed.
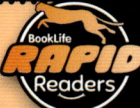

MARLIN
The fastest animals under water, marlins will be blasting through their journey.

FALCON
The fastest animals in the air, falcons will be flying at top speed as they tear through the skies.